Soul Portrait

Improve Your Quality of Life by Making Aging Personal

by Sally Zuck McBain

Cover Photos by: "Oh Shoot" photography by Jan, *The Dalles, Oregon*

First published by Dog Ear Publishing
4010 W. 86th Street, Ste H
Indianapolis, IN 46268
www.dogearpublishing.net

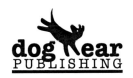

ISBN: 978-1-4575-0792-2

This book is printed on acid-free paper.

Printed in the United States of America

In Memoriam

Soul Portrait is dedicated to the memory of my parents, Clark and Aleta Zuck. Theirs was a legacy of love.

Table of Contents

Acknowledgments

Many people have blessed *Soul Portrait*'s journey, and I am grateful to each and every one. With their encouragement, editing skills, emotional support, and shared experiences, individuals of all ages and from all walks of life contributed to its growth and development over the last ten years.

Among the first to read *Soul Portrait* were Carole Anderson, Kimberly and Randy Gillenwater, Christine Jacobson, Joy and Bill Mallonee, Rhonda Schutz, Bill Barnett, and Deborah Berger. Their belief in *Soul Portrait* has sustained me and strengthened my resolve to make aging personal.

Family therapist, Satsuki Ina, was my favorite professor at the University of Oregon. She led her graduate-level classes through the complex world of families and aging with a spark that still burns in me 26 years later. Dr. Ina's enthusiasm for *Soul Portrait* has been a gift, one which honors me in more ways than I could ever express.

For over thirty years, tireless relatives and caregivers have shared their frustrations, joys, laughter, and tears with me. These individuals are the backbone of the elder care system; they continue to inspire me over and over again with their courage and dedication.

Several people participated in a focus group before I published *Soul Portrait*. While *Soul Portrait* was written with elders and families in mind, they reminded me that taking an introspective look at one's life is beneficial for an adult of any age. Scott McKay, Judy Merrill, Lucile and Jim Torgerson, Lyn Dalton, Ron Nelson, and Jeanne Hillis offered more than their time, personal stories, and helpful suggestions; they injected new life into *Soul Portrait*.

Erie, Pennsylvania native, Ted Trampenau, deserves special notice in *Soul Portrait*. He did not learn of *Soul Portrait* until after his wife died, at which point he said, "I lived your book with my Nancy." He was by his wife's side every day, all day, for three years. During that time, he made sure everyone in the nursing facility knew the Nancy he knew. I am pleased to include Ted's letter to men in *Soul Portrait*.

I could not have written *Soul Portrait* without the input and steadfast support of my husband, Ken. Because of his 40-year career in health care administration, he knows how important it is to make aging personal.

Finally, there is one person to whom I attribute my choice of aging as a life work. She was my predecessor and adviser when I started out in 1980 as in-home care supervisor for an area agency on aging. In just a few weeks, not only did she show me what it takes to be a compassionate professional, Suzanne Madden helped me lay the foundation upon which I built my career.

Introduction

My father was a farmer, so it was no surprise when he announced, "If the time comes I can't take care of myself, take me out behind the barn and shoot me. Just plow me under; it'll be easier and a lot cheaper." Most families would be mortified to hear a parent talk like this, but we knew he was trying to make light of something that frightened him more and more as he got older.

Dad was typical of elders who do not want to be a burden on others; but just as important to him was maintaining his independence. All it takes is a stroll down the halls of a nursing home and we can relate to his fear of not being in control of his life. Helpless older and disabled adults sit in the halls or lie in bed in lonely silence, waiting for a nurse's aide to accompany them to the bathroom, take them to the showers, or wheel them to a meal.

Though lying in a hospital or nursing home bed is not an inevitable outcome of aging, it grows more possible as we age. Whether we are recuperating in a facility for a few weeks or in our own home receiving care, someday our lives could be in the hands of someone else.

During most of my career, I worked with older people who needed help but were living independently at home. Later, when I served as admissions coordinator for a skilled nursing facility, I was exposed to adults who were totally dependent on others for their survival. One such woman stands out in my mind. Her name was Maria.

Every day, on my way to or from a resident's room, I encountered Maria in her wheelchair, staring out the dining room window. I knew she could not speak because of a recent stroke, but I was determined to try to communicate with her.

One morning I got down on my knees beside Maria's wheelchair and began to talk about how lovely the birds sounded after a long winter's silence. I looked out the window with her, pointing at flowering trees and song birds she could see from where she sat. I found it easy to identify with her love of Nature.

It was a brief encounter, and with the exception of what I thought was her attempt at a smile, nothing I said seemed to strike a familiar chord with her. On the way back to my office I began to wonder if I had made too many assumptions about Maria. I thought she was doing what I would do; I would be wishing I were sitting under a tree, holding out a handful of bird seed for the nearest chickadee. I wanted to learn more about Maria, so I headed for the nurses' station to see what they knew about her.

One of the nurses thought Maria sat at the window every day so she could watch for her son. Another assumed she was waiting for lunch to be served. An aide remarked, "I usually put her there after we get her dressed for the day. I thought she'd like to be near all the activity instead of in her room." Obviously, they didn't know any more about Maria than I did.

Whenever I passed Maria at the window, I wondered who she was and what she was thinking. What did she enjoy about life? What were her fears? In what or whom did she believe? What sustained her in hard times? How could we satisfy some of her emotional and spiritual needs?

There was no way to know the answers to these questions without the help of her children or an intimate friend. That would be difficult, since Maria's son came by infrequently and she had no other visitors. But even if she had, the questions are personal, and Maria may not have shared such things with someone else.

I found myself wishing she had written something about herself, a personal profile of sorts, one that included information we could use to provide her with individualized attention. But Maria was a stranger to us, and because we knew nothing about her, we could not tend to her deepest needs – her soul needs.

We offered good care, but it was the same standard nursing and personal care we gave to all our residents. Had we known more about Maria, we could have provided her with an atmosphere better attuned to her individuality, and by doing so, improved her quality of life.

I pictured myself in Maria's shoes, unable to tell my caregivers who I am and what I need or want. Not only would I be frustrated and scared, I might feel like giving up right then and there. I wondered how I could affect the care given to me by someone else so I would thrive rather than simply exist.

The challenge before me was to come up with a way we can share the deepest part of ourselves while we are still able. My response to this challenge is an account of who we are at the most basic level, a snapshot of our soul, or as I'm calling it, *Soul Portrait*.

How to Use *Soul Portrait*

I wrote *Soul Portrait* to bring attention to the need for more personalized health care. As a MAP (Making Aging Personal) to the self, one which can be shared with others, it opens the road to dignity, individuality, empathy, and respect. Although I have written *Soul Portrait* within the context of aging and dependency, it can be used by anyone who wants to think more deeply about who they are and what life means to them.

A completed *Soul Portrait* makes a great gift to present to family members who wish to know more about us. Our name is on the family tree, but who is the person behind that name? In this electronic age of fast-paced access to information, *Soul Portrait* encourages us to slow down and reach out to those we love. It helps us talk about sensitive issues, understand one another, and make life-long soul connections.

Soul Portrait can provide comfort as we navigate our way through the maze of today's health care system. While we cope with acute and chronic illness, rising costs of care, and the many professionals who pass in and out of our lives, it gets more difficult to stay connected to self and soul without some support. The best way to do that is to make our aging personal. We can contribute to our current peace of mind and future well-being by letting others know who we are beneath the surface, so they can advocate for us when and if we cannot advocate for ourselves.

For individuals who are reticent to discuss their aging and possible dependency, *Soul Portrait* is a non-threatening way to open up channels of communication. *Soul Portrait* encourages thoughtful answers and joint problem-solving. It can be a painless first step in guiding families though discussions about the future. Questions may come up, such as, "Where do you want to live if you can't take care of yourself?" If the answer is, "with my oldest son", now is the time to find out if that is realistic. The oldest son and his wife may already have their eyes on the local assisted living facility.

By openly sharing who we are, we encourage medical personnel, social workers, spiritual advisers, support staff, volunteers, and caregivers to look beyond what they see and what they assume about us. Physical care requires sensitivity, skill, patience, and attention to human dignity; but it is not the same as caring for the soul. We need both components of care in order to receive the best care possible.

To Future *Soul Portrait* Authors

The following topics, with whatever additions you make, will soon become your *Soul Portrait*. They are arranged alphabetically so someone else can find them at a moment's notice. Each one includes an excerpt from my own *Soul Portrait*, along with a question or two to get you started. I have left space on your title page for a current photograph of yourself; it will immediately remind busy providers they are watching over the life of a person who has an identity beyond a name, diagnosis, and treatment plan.

You can design your *Soul Portrait* in several ways: writing, sketching, cutting and pasting, or dictating your thoughts to someone else who will write for you. My personal copy of *Soul Portrait* is a combination of my writing and pictures I gathered from magazines – a collage with words. I did it that way to entice others to look a little closer at who I am; one picture of a piece of chocolate cake in the <u>Comfort</u> section says a lot.

Writing is the primary way I express myself, yet it doesn't always come easily to me; it took me years to find my own voice. My breakthrough came when I realized the best writing comes from the heart. Trust what comes out, what you feel, and what you need to express. You can make lists, write where your thoughts take you, or simply enter a couple key words under a topic. Make it as simple or detailed as you wish. If you choose the latter approach, you may wish to highlight key words or thoughts so caregivers can quickly see what you want them to know.

After you have read *Soul Portrait*, I suggest you close it for a while and think about what and how you want to share. Give your mind time to settle into the purpose of *Soul Portrait*. Ideas will bubble up naturally as you go about your day, and you may want to record them so you don't forget. Having a separate notebook will help you through this phase, but that is your choice. You may want to begin writing, drawing, or cutting and pasting the moment you open *Soul Portrait*.

Some people type on a computer and print out their topics to place in a binder of their own making. Others write in the book itself; still others write by hand on notebook paper. Do what makes you comfortable. If you fly model airplanes, include a photo of your favorite and explain how you got interested in flying. If you love to sew, attach a swatch of your favorite fabric or a picture of your daughter in the wedding dress you made. If you volunteer for a special charity, write about how and why you chose that particular one. Whatever you decide to do, the point of *Soul Portrait* is to share with others who you are.

What you write today could change with the passage of time. If you are typing your *Soul Portrait* on the computer, topics are easily modified. If you are doing your *Soul Portrait* by long-hand, write the date at the top of your new entry, indicating that things have changed. Your *Soul Portrait* may end up being a work-in-progress, one which reveals an ever-expressive side of yourself.

If you can no longer write due to a disability, you may wish to put your thoughts on a recorder; but you will eventually need to get help entering your comments on the page so your care providers can immediately go to a particular topic.

There will be aides, nurses, and physicians who won't have time to look at your *Soul Portrait*. With a growing shortage of providers, ever-changing rules and regulations, and swelling numbers of people over the age of 65, professionals are stretched to the limit. That doesn't mean your *Soul Portrait* won't be appreciated and used; it will. If a family member, neighbor, or friend knows you have it and where you keep it, they can use it to advocate for you. The more they know about you, the more effective their advocacy.

Soul Portrait can improve your quality of life and the care you receive, whether you are at the doctor's office, have been hospitalized, live at home, or reside in a group or congregate setting. If you have recently been diagnosed with Alzheimer's disease or a related disorder, now is the time to contribute to your own well-being and sense of familiarity by making your *Soul Portrait*. The soul-needs you share now may stimulate recognition and bring you comfort later.

I wish you well in your process of introspection and sharing. You may never need *Soul Portrait* for health care purposes, but you will be leaving a legacy of the best kind to those who know and love you. There can be no better gift.

A Letter to Men

Gentlemen:

You may think *Soul Portrait* is just for women, but it's for you, too. For instance, you can describe your love of the outdoors on the <u>Activities Page</u>: hunting, fishing, skiing, camping, golfing, and more. Write about the sports you follow, your likes and dislikes, your hobbies, and favorite things to do with family and friends. I enjoy talking about airplanes and flying, and spending time with my daughters.

Some men may be reluctant to admit they need help to plan in advance for their future health care needs. Maybe you planned for a comfortable retirement and drew up your will. Now, with the guidance of your *Soul Portrait*, you can prepare for a different facet of your life, for the day you may be completely dependent on someone else to take care of you.

Soul Portrait covers a broad range of topics that will help caregivers see you as a whole person. The care you receive will reflect this special knowledge should you be unable to convey your concerns and desires directly; and it can improve your life.

For three years until her death on February 25, 2010, my wife, Nancy, was a resident at St. Mary's nursing home in Erie, PA. I lived *Soul Portrait* with her, and as a result, everyone knew Nancy as a whole person, a woman with a personality and an interesting life-story. Because of this, she received the best care possible.

It will be well worth your time to go through the entire book like I did, and then produce your own *Soul Portrait*. I wish you good health and a long and fruitful life.

Sincerely,
Ted Trampenau

My Soul Portrait

by

_____

(your photograph)

Activities

I love to bake, knit, write, and paint with watercolors. Usually, I do something active every day, like walking or yoga. Sitting still is a challenge for me. I know I may not be able to do these things someday, but please don't try to substitute TV for real activity. If I have to sit in front of something, I'd much rather sit in front of a picture window or a tank full of colorful fish.

What activities do you enjoy? Do you have a favorite hobby or sport?

Animal Friends

My golden retriever's name is Molly. She's the sweetest dog I ever had, and she is getting old. I don't know what life will be like without her, so I'm trying to enjoy every moment. I'm also trying not to let her hear me complain about her hair all over the place. I'm convinced animals know much more than they let on. I've had cats, too, but I decided dogs are easier to talk to; and I do a lot of talking.

Do you have a favorite pet? What role have animals played in your life?

Beliefs

I believe God is love – love that resides in each and every one of us. I believe anger is a cover-up for fear. I believe we should get in the habit of telling others what we like about them; and I believe 'I love you' should be unconditional and not based on how happy someone else makes us at any given time.

In what or whom do you believe? How have these beliefs shaped your life?

Clothing

If I'm recuperating from an illness and too weak to get out of bed, I would appreciate an attractive bed jacket to cheer me up. There is nothing more depressing than wearing a nightgown all day long. I have a favorite sweater I wear when I'm chilly. It's a red one I knit many years ago. It's not too heavy, and the multicolored buttons cheer me up.

How do you like to dress? Do you have a special garment you can't live without?

Color

Yellow energizes me: I perk up at the sight of yellow ribbons, yellow tulips, and yellow shadows cast by the bright morning sun. Green relaxes me: I feel my blood pressure go down when I walk in green grass, look into green eyes, and imagine myself floating down a green river. Red is my soul color: I love red leaves, red skies, red soil, and red birds.

What are your favorite colors? Do they mean something special to you?

Comfort

Inspirational quotes have always provided me with comfort during difficult times. One of my favorites is, "Be still and know that I am God." Meditative breathing helps, too, along with prayers for guidance and patience. Nature is the one stable influence in my life that always soothes me. If I need immediate comfort, however, a piece of very rich, very chocolate cake will do.

What comforts you? Do you go to a special place or person for comfort?

Conversation

I love a good chat. I like to talk about American history, the places I've lived and traveled, and the books I've read or movies I've seen. I'm interested in many things – philosophy, current events, and the arts. I'm also intrigued by stories others have to tell.

What do you like to talk about? Is there a special topic that can hold your interest for hours?

Distractions

There are several sounds that drive me nuts and keep me from concentrating on my writing or reading. I can't stand loud TV's and booming rock music, the sound of heavy construction equipment, barking dogs, and the sawing down of trees. Because there will always be distracting noises, I put on my headset and listen to beautiful music instead.

What annoys you so much it distracts you from doing other things?

Education

I graduated from college in 1969 with a BA in sociology; but as much as I value my formal education, I have learned just as much from the people around me. Of course, like everyone else, I got an advanced degree from the school of hard-knocks and mistakes. The biggest lessons I learned came out of divorce and many years alone. Mostly, I learned about myself.

How did you learn what you know today? What was your greatest lesson?

Family Wisdom

The wisdom I inherited came from my father. It was, "Always put yourself in the other guy's shoes." It has never failed me; that advice helped me become more understanding and less judgmental of other people. If we all did more of that, the world would be a better place.

Did a family member (or someone else) share something wise with you? How did it impact your life?

Fear

I'm afraid of being closed in. I've struggled with my claustrophobia for years, so if I become agitated and can't tell you what's wrong, that may be the reason. It keeps me from flying or being in a small area filled with people. I like to know where exits are if I'm in a strange place. I'm also afraid of German shepherds because one lunged at me a few years back and took a piece out of my jacket.

What are you afraid of? How does that fear affect your life?

Feelings

I wear my feelings on my sleeve. When I'm happy, I get giddy. When I'm sad, I cry. When I'm angry, I can get snippy; but most of the time I come out talking. Rarely do I sulk or hold in how I feel. I talk about feelings as readily as some people talk about the weather, mainly because I think feelings (and how we express them) provide important clues to who we are.

How do you express your feelings? Do you tend to hold them in or share them?

Flowers

"If I had but two loaves of bread, I would sell one and buy hyacinths, for they would feed my soul." This quote from the Koran reflects my feelings. The smell and intricate detail of a blossom bring me joy. My studio walls are covered with my photos and painting of flowers. Because of their sweet scents, my favorites are lilacs, sweet peas, gardenias, and freesia.

What are your favorite flowers? Do you have a garden?

Food

With the exception of slimy oysters, I can't think of anything I won't eat. Mealtime is a special time, a time to savor incredible flavors and be grateful for all I have. Among my favorite choices are poached eggs on toast, anything Greek or Mexican, Monte Cristo sandwiches, and grilled salmon or chicken. I enjoy red wine, and I love fruit pie and lemon or chocolate cake.

What do you like to eat? What foods do you dislike?

Forgiveness

Before I could forgive others or ask for their forgiveness, I had to learn how to forgive myself. Over the years, I've been blessed by the forgiveness of loved ones and have tried to be generous with my own. When something goes wrong in a relationship and I can identify my sensitivities and understand theirs, forgiveness is easy.

Are you generous with your forgiveness? Do you need the forgiveness of someone in your life?

Gratitude

I often write in a journal about all the things I'm grateful for, like the feel of a ray of sun on my face, a loon's call, or the sight of a soaring red-tailed hawk. Not a day goes by I don't feel grateful for something in Nature; I love being able to experience all these wonders. I also write about the gift of someone's love. I am grateful for my family and friends, and I try to tell them often how much they mean to me.

For what and whom are you grateful? How do you express your gratitude?

Happiness

I'm happiest when I'm in my studio, creating something and looking out on rocks, pines, and scrub oaks. Happiness is coming up with the perfect line to end a poem, sketching an animal that looks like the real thing, and making greeting cards with my photographs. I'm also happy when I'm spending quality time with people I love.

What makes you happy? Where or with whom are you most happy?

Holidays and Celebrations

I avoided holidays when I was divorced and living alone. I had a small artificial tree that brought solace, but not the mood to celebrate. Now, Christmas is one of my favorite occasions. I still have that little tree decked out in colored lights, and I still decorate it with small treasures of the past. All the big Christmas trees in the world can't take the place of my sweet little tree.

What do you like to celebrate? How do you celebrate?

Hopes, Prayers, and Dreams

I dream of a peace-filled, hunger-free, environmentally-stable planet. I pray for full, healthy, violent-free lives for all the world's children. I dream of the things I want to create into my old age, and I hope I can stay active for many years to come. Most of all, I hope and pray I am never a burden on my children.

What are your hopes and dreams?

Humor

I love a good laugh. I have scrapbooks filled with my favorite cartoons, like Charles Schulz's *Peanuts*, Jim Unger's *Herman*, and Gary Larson's *The Far Side*. I can watch a funny movie several times; and the same goes for sitcoms like *Friends* and *Seinfeld*. I don't care for slapstick humor or jokes that poke fun at other people.

What makes you laugh? What kind of humor offends you?

Identity

For years, I tried to figure out who I am. Mostly, I think of myself as an introvert with a lot of creative energy. When my elder son was in 10th grade, he wrote a poem that described me as, "A person, a woman, a worker, an administrator, a doer, an achiever, a write, a creator, a confidant, a friend. But most of all – a mom."

How would you identify yourself? How might someone else identify you?

Idiosyncrasies

I like lemon in iced tea and milk in hot tea. I like to have two pillows for my head when I'm sleeping, and I prefer a couple blankets rather than an electric blanket in the winter. I don't like air conditioning that is so cold I need a wool jacket; in all kinds of weather, I like to crack open a window so I can get some fresh air. Most of all, I dislike bright lights with a passion.

What makes you unique? What special things do you need for your physical comfort?

Loss

The biggest loss of my life was the death of my parents four months apart. It took me two years to adjust to their being gone; it seemed my grief would never end. One never stops being a daughter, but it's different now. I didn't fully appreciate all they did for me. I hope there is a life after this one so I can thank them again – this time, as a daughter who knows a whole lot more about being a parent.

Did you suffer a loss that changed your life? How did it change you?

Love, Honor, and Respect

I feel loved when someone brings me flowers, sends me a card for no reason, or gives me something they made with their own hands. I know I'm being honored when another person validates my feelings instead of brushing them aside; and I know I'm respected when someone tells me the truth instead of glossing over or avoiding it.

How do you know when you are being loved, honored, and respected?

Memories

I have memories I'd rather forget, but that makes it easier to focus on the good ones. Some of my best memories come from my childhood; it was great living on a farm. Later, I added memories of my own children and the beautiful places I've lived. One thing I'll never forget happened when I was a harried young mom: our garbage collector reached down from the cab of the dump truck and handed me a rose.

What memories do you treasure?

Music

I need a lot of silence, but I can't live without music. On the radio, I search out classical and Celtic compositions. If I have my headphones on with my favorites, many of which are themes from movies, I can transport myself to a peaceful place. I used to play the piano, and its sound is one of my favorites, along with that of a cello.

What music do you enjoy?   Do you play an instrument or sing?

Nature

If I'm ever confined to bed, I hope I can see a tree or two. It will remind me of the trees I loved when I was a child: maple trees that dropped mounds of burnt orange and gold leaves, the huge spruce tree under whose drooping boughs I could hide, and the fruit trees from our orchard that yielded the best apples and plums ever consumed by a little girl. Nature is so much a part of my life, I always write it with the capital letter, 'N'.

Do you feel a connection with Nature? What gives you a sense of awe?

Occupation

My working life began when I was a teenager and sold fresh turkey products in one of my father's stores. Right out of college, I taught pre-school and kindergarten; and after my sons were born, I enjoyed being a mother and homemaker. My career in the field of aging began when the boys were in school, and I've been rewarded by that choice over and over again.

What kinds of jobs have you had? Did you serve in the armed forces or another branch of public service?

Outlook

I like to think of the glass as half full, but I also inherited a worry-gene from my mother, who inherited it from her mother. I have to remind myself to take a day at a time and see life as a series of blessings rather than potential problems. I'm cheerful most of the time, and for that, I thank my dad. He had a good disposition and would often say, "Ain't life grand?"

How would you describe your outlook on life?

Passion

My definition of passion is something you not only love to do, you have to do it. I have to create, whether with a pen, paint brush, knitting needles, or my 40-year-old hand-mixer. The act of creating connects me with the deepest part of myself and gives me a sense of purpose and joy.

What are your passions?

Personality

I'm emotional, impatient, open, sincere, and sentimental. I can be loud and playful when I get excited or think something is funny. Essential to my well-being is my need to be alone; I'm a classic introvert. While I enjoy being around other people, the experience takes a lot of my energy and I need to balance it with a good measure of quiet solitude.

How would you describe your personality?

Pet Peeves

I get irritated with people who use two parking spaces for their car, neighbors who let their dogs run loose, and individuals who throw trash from their moving vehicle. In a nutshell, it bothers me when people don't consider how their actions affect the rest of us.

What are your pet peeves?

Pride

Pride is a lot of things to me. I was reared to be humble, but every now and then, I puff up with pride at a painting I've done or a sweater I've knitted. I'm proud of my sons and who they have become. I'm proud of my independent nature and my ability to take care of myself when I have to, even though it gets in the way of my asking for help when I could really use it. I'm working on that.

What does the word 'pride' mean to you? Have you done something that makes you proud of yourself?

Reading Preferences

Books and magazines have always been a big part of my life. I love poetry by Rilke, Rumi, and Mary Oliver. I also enjoy the writing of Wallace Stegner; he and Wendell Berry are two of my favorite authors. If I'm tired and don't feel like reading a book, I enjoy the mindless exercise of flipping through fashion magazines and complaining about the cost of wrinkle creams and shoes.

What do you like to read?

Religion and Spirituality

I'm a solitary worshiper. I find God in doing the supper dishes or knitting a pair of socks. I see God in the sunset or a child's face. If I am in need of spiritual inspiration or last words, I would prefer the services of someone who believes the best practice of all is unconditional love.

What would you like to share about your religion or spirituality?

Routines and Rituals

Routines keep me grounded, and rituals help me live a spiritual life. When I get up, I pour my coffee (darkest roast I can buy) and go into my studio to read and write. A couple hours later, I'm ready for a walk. In the afternoon, after a nap, I meditate and then paint. Around 5 p.m. wine hour caps off a productive day. I love the stability routines offer, but I always try to stay flexible.

What routines and rituals do you follow?

Seasons

My favorite season is autumn. Maybe it's a throw-back from my school days, but it marks the beginning of my year. Autumn is when I make my resolutions, set up my new year's calendar, and start planning projects. The cool air, soft light, and changing colors thrill and inspire me. With the arrival of September, I make sure my camera is charged up and ready to shoot.

What is your favorite season? Why?

Smells

Smells bring back memories. I love the fragrance of gardenia, which my college roommate and I wore all the time. Calming lavender reminds me of my maternal grandmother; and hot moist soil takes me back 60 years to the steamy greenhouses my family owned. As for bad smells, I cringe when a skunk passes by the house at night, because I remember all too well the time our golden retriever met up with one.

What are your favorite smells? What smells are offensive to you?

Special Interests

I have a special interest in wild things. I'm not a scientist by any stretch; but I pay close attention to local animals. My favorites are coyotes, bison, owls, song birds, loons, and mountain goats. Because I have lived in so many different places, each of these animals has crossed my path at one time or another.

What are your special interests?

Surroundings

I'm surrounded by books and magazines, photographs of my family, a good radio/CD player, art supplies, and items from nature. I used to have a lot of plants, but I had to give most of them away when we moved from Pennsylvania to Oregon. Now, I like to buy fresh flowers.

What items do you like to have around you?

Touch

I love to get bear hugs from special people, and I groan with delight when my husband rubs my feet and legs at night. I like the way a book feels in my hand, and how the textures and shapes of smooth stones, tree bark, and sea shells remind me of times at the shore or in the woods.

How do you feel about being touched? What textures appeal to you?

Travel

I have lived in, and traveled through, much of the United States and parts of Canada. My favorite home has always been the Columbia River Gorge. My favorite vacation spots are the Grand Tetons, Sedona, the Sonoran desert, and the rocky Oregon coast. I was born on the shores of Lake Erie, but I'm a westerner at heart.

Where have you lived and traveled? Do you have a favorite vacation spot?

Truth

The only time I accept a half-truth is when it comes to my vanity. If I ask someone, "How do I look?", I won't mind a little embellishment. But if I have an illness that cannot be treated or healed, I want to know. There will be things needing to be said, and business needing to be done. When it comes to telling the truth, I'm getting better at that with age.

How do you feel about being told the truth? Are you able to tell the truth when it's necessary?

Values

The three values I hold most dear are unconditional love, self-resect, and non-judgment. Each day, I try to live by them. When I'm in doubt about how to react to someone else, I always run those values through my mind. Do I love without expectations? Am I being true to myself when I express an opinion or desire? Do I refrain from making judgments about others? If I hesitate, I know I have some work to do.

What values do you try to live by?

Vanity

I admit to being vain; but the older I get, the less preoccupied I am with the way I look. I try to focus on things that matter to me, like writing and painting. I still care about my appearance though, and would appreciate someone putting some color on my cheeks and trimming the hairs on my chin if I can't do it. I also want to be told when I have a blob of something from lunch on my blouse.

Are you vain about certain things?

Additional Thoughts

Reflections

Ten years have passed since the birth of *Soul Portrait*. Its theme – making aging personal – holds even more meaning for me now, as I reflect on my mother's last days.

In the span of a year and a half, Mother was admitted to a nursing home five different times. It was during those stays that I got to know who she was beyond her role as a parent. With *Soul Portrait* as my guide, I used our time together to learn more about her. She had always been a private person, the product of a generation that did not readily share thoughts and feelings; it wasn't appropriate to be centered on self. Relating family stories and history was more acceptable than talking about personal dreams, fears, or joys.

Always one to dig further for personal truths and connection, I wanted to form a deeper bond with my mother. She knew almost everything there was to know about me, her blunt and open-book third child. Now, I wanted our precious time together to be about her, not about her four children, my father, or her grandchildren. *Soul Portrait* helped me re-direct her back to herself.

In early December 2005, she was in the nursing home for the last time. She had suffered a stroke and could not speak. I was with her most of the week before she died, working alongside aides and Hospice nurses to keep her comfortable. My solace came in knowing exactly what music fed her soul, how she liked her covers tucked up under her chin, how she wanted to hide her disheveled hair-do with a stylish turban, and when she needed to be alone more than she needed visitors. I knew what made her anxious and what made her smile. I knew the joys she surely clung to as she took her last breath. And I knew she was not afraid to die.

People tell me they have used *Soul Portrait* to confront issues that arise with aging, illness, dementia, dependence, and dying. These turning points have the potential to bring us closer to one another, magnify our similarities, and encourage forgiveness, understanding, and respect. At the same time, we are blessed by the little things that make each of us unique. *Soul Portrait* is one way to express our individuality, while at the same time, build on the foundation which connects us all.

Afterword

It was 1998 when I met Dan, a 72-year-old resident in the brand new nursing home where I worked as admissions coordinator. Dan had suffered a stroke, and along with other functioning, he lost his ability to form most words and make sentences.

Every day when the weather was comfortable, Dan wheeled himself out to the veranda at the entryway to the facility. There, he could greet visitors and watch the traffic.

One morning, I was on my way into work when I decided to spend a few minutes with him. As soon as I sat down beside Dan, a fire truck passed in front of us. He became animated, so I asked him if he liked fire trucks. Dan responded with a loud, "Why, yesss!!' He attempted to say more, and I tried to help him by asking other questions that would elicit another enthusiastic response, but to no avail.

Later that day, a fellow resident told me Dan had been a fireman. Because I didn't know this, I missed the opportunity to talk to him about something with which he identified, something that had been a big part of his life.

My friend Trish is lying in a nursing home bed today, suffering from the end stages of multiple sclerosis. Her two children live in the surrounding area, but they lead busy lives and can't visit on a regular basis.

Trish has been in this nursing facility for over twelve years. I lived in another state all that time, so when I moved back, I went to see her. She did not remember me and she could not speak without getting tired, so I did most of the talking.

I stayed an hour with Trish, telling her about our good times together and watching her eyes light up with recognition every now and then. On my way out, I stopped at the nurses' station to ask several questions about her early diagnosis and progression of the disease. I also asked if they knew how talented, feisty, and creative Trish had been in the old days, or how she kept a vegetable garden and canned specialties for her friends. I wondered if they knew she cooked incredible meals in a tiny kitchen, dressed like a model on a Salvation Army budget, and reared two small children on her own after her husband died from cancer.

They had not known any of this; in fact, staff had turned over several times since Trish was admitted, losing any history the earlier nurses and aides might have known about her.

The moment Trish entered the care facility, she became a patient; and the wholeness of her life was lost. Without being able to weave threads of the past into the current fabric of her life, staff would never know the Trish I knew – the confident, fiercely independent and in-control Trish I admired. Had they known more about her, her caregivers might have understood her anger and defiance at the onset of her illness.

Personal connections are at the heart of good health care, but because of many factors, some of which I mentioned earlier, they are often at the bottom of the list of priorities. Advocates play a critical role in making aging personal, and *Soul Portrait* can help them. Because topics are easy to find, *Soul Portrait* gives them information at a glance. One or two facts about our life can personalize an otherwise frightening and intimidating experience.

Soul Portrait is our MAP to a higher quality of life, one that can be followed easily by family, friends, and health care providers. Making aging personal is the only way to get answers to the question, "Who are you?" Whether it is used now or saved for the future, *Soul Portrait* brings the answers to life.

About the Author

Sally Zuck McBain began her work with older adults in 1980, serving as homemaker supervisor for 'Oregon Project Independence', a state-funded in-home care program for older adults. Following that experience, she directed a five-county area agency on aging in Oregon, coordinated admissions to a 120-bed nursing facility in Nevada, and served as the founding executive director of the Wyoming Gerontological Association.

As her interest in the field of gerontology developed, Sally became aware of the need to get more information about aging out to older adults and their families. She led workshops, spoke to community groups about available resources, wrote a bi-monthly column on aging for several Oregon newspapers, hosted weekly radio programs, and facilitated caregiver and grief support groups.

Sally continued her studies by doing graduate-level work in gerontology at the University of Oregon, and attending the National Leadership Institute on Aging in Denver, Colorado, under the direction of the late Dale Neugarten.

CPSIA information can be obtained at www.ICGtesting.com
Printed in the USA
LVOW112055090312

272454LV00002B/1/P